AND OTHER
WEIGHTY ISSUES

A GIRL CODE BOOK

CATHY HAMILTON

Andrews McMeel Publishing

Kansas City

DIETING AND OTHER WEIGHTY ISSUES

copyright © 2001 by Ms. Communications.
All rights reserved. Printed in the United States
of America. No part of this book may be used
or reproduced in any manner whatsoever without
written permission except in the case of reprints
in the context of reviews. For information,
write Andrews McMeel Publishing,
an Andrews McMeel Universal company,
4520 Main Street, Kansas City, Missouri 64111.

01 02 03 04 05 BIN 10 9 8 7 6 5 4 3 2 1

ISBN: 0-7407-1862-2

Library of Congress Control Number:
2001089270

Attention: Schools and Businesses

Andrews McMeel books are available at quantity discounts with
bulk purchase for educational, business, or sales promotional
use. For information, please write to: Special Sales Department,
Andrews McMeel Publishing, 4520 Main Street,
Kansas City, Missouri 64111.

CONTENTS

RULES AND RATIONALIZATIONS
1

THE BUDDY SYSTEM
19

BOTTOM LINES
31

SHOPPING STRATEGIES
37

BINGE BYLAWS
51

THE NAKED TRUTH
(OR FULL DIS-CLOTHES-URE)
71

EXERCISING YOUR RIGHTS
77

MIRRORS, SCALES, AND OTHER
DISTORTIONS OF NATURE
83

RULES
AND
RATIONALI-
ZATIONS

—⚀—

If you *think* you're big-boned, you *are* big-boned.

Never ask a man "Do I look fat?" as if you expect an honest answer.

No man has the right to know how much you weigh, except your physician and lifeboat captain.

This includes boyfriends and husbands.

When a fellow girl asks "Do I look fat?" the best answer is "You look great!"

If you think your metabolism is slow, it *is* slow.

It is never appropriate to make the comment "I am so fat!" if:

You are a size 10 or smaller.

You are the exact same size or smaller than any girl in the room.

You are a Victoria's Secret model or someone with similar proportions.

You used to be fat but have recently lost a significant amount of weight.

Never, *ever* ask a woman "When are you due?" unless you're *sure* she's pregnant!

*Author's note:
Once, while wearing a baggy jumper, I was asked this question by an acquaintance of my mother's. When I explained that I was not, in fact, pregnant, the woman was mortified. Her face turned the color of paprika and she apologized no less than nine times. Her attempts at atonement were worse than the original remark, which is why I also recommend . . .*

If someone asks you "When are you due?" and you are *not*, in fact, pregnant, simply reply: "Any minute now!" Save yourself the aggravation.

You are *not* what you eat.

How ridiculous is that? I mean, if that were true, we'd all be nothing but big vats of pasta alfredo.

You can reasonably attribute five pounds of your weight at any given time to "water retention."

Before your period, ten to fifteen pounds is acceptable.

You may understate your weight by up to twenty-five pounds on your driver's license in most states without raising an eyebrow.

Any more and you're pushing your luck.

A woman is never expected to tell the truth about her weight.

Never ask another woman "How much do you weigh?" unless you are a doctor, nurse, anesthesiologist, or lifeboat captain.

If you hang out with fatter people, you will look thinner.

This is particularly true by the pool or on the beach.

(Warning: Hanging out with the fatties too often could give you a false sense of security and lead to overeating.)

Never date a man with thinner arms than yours.

Author's note:
My rule used to be "never date a man with thinner thighs *than yours" until I realized I had eliminated 90 percent of the eligible men in the free world.*

Keep plenty of healthy snacks around the house and office.

Even if you never touch them, you'll give others the impression that you're trying.

THE
BUDDY
SYSTEM

———♀———

It is never acceptable to sabotage a fellow girl's diet, even if you desperately want someone to binge with.

It's a given that when you lose weight, others will be jealous and try to sabotage you.

Note: These people are not your true friends.

When a girl tells you how much weight she's lost, don't question the amount. Believe her and cheer for every pound.

When you know a girl has been dieting seriously for more than two weeks, tell her she looks skinnier . . . even if she doesn't!

When a fellow girl has lost a significant amount of weight, applaud her efforts like you'd want her to celebrate with you.

When a girlfriend is dieting, don't eat ice cream, chocolate, or other tempting foods in front of her.

But if you must (say, like at a wedding), don't act like you're enjoying it. Tell her it's the worst cake you ever had.

When you are on a diet, you are not required to cook a separate meal for the nondieting members of your household.

Let the skinny freaks fend for themselves.

It is never advisable to start a weight-loss competition with a girlfriend.

*It's a no-win situation.
No matter which one of you loses more, the other will lose less.
So you both lose.*

Never *ever* compete in a weight-loss contest with a man.

Men can lose ten pounds in three days just by giving up beer. Dieting is aggravating enough . . . who needs that?

There is nothing more obnoxious than a person who has lost a significant amount of weight and thinks she has suddenly become the calorie police.

If you're going to cheat, go all the way.

Don't waste a perfectly good binge on something stupid like a Twinkie when, for the same amount of guilt, a crème brûlée is MUCH more satisfying.

THE BOTTOM LINE

♀

Never ask a man
"Does my butt look big?"
and expect an answer you
can live with.

Visible panty lines add ten pounds.

Avoid them at all costs.

Friends don't let friends wear fanny packs.

Hip hugger jeans were designed for women with no hips.

Only one out of 99 women can get away with wearing a thong.

Chances are, you're not one of them.

SHOPPING STRATEGIES

───♀───

Never shop with girls who are significantly skinnier than you. A good rule of thumb is to practice departmental segregation.

Juniors should not shop with Misses.

Misses should not shop with Women's.

Petites should not shop with Talls, etc.

When shopping for swimsuits, always go solo.

If someone asks what size you are, it is appropriate to answer with the lowest size in your closet that you can still squeeze into.

If a girl asks you if an outfit makes her look fat, tell her the truth gently. Say "I think you could find something more flattering," or "It doesn't seem to hang very well on you."

You'd want her to do the same for you.

Never tell a fellow girl that something doesn't look good on her, then turn around and buy it for yourself.

Designer clothes almost always run larger than knock-offs.

Sometimes, it's worth spending the extra money to say you wear a 10.

When in doubt,
buy the larger size.

*This is especially true
for swimsuits.*

The outfit will never look as fabulous on you as it does on the mannequin.

Keep in mind, the typical mannequin is over five foot ten tall and measures 34-24-35.

Tube tops, bicycle shorts, white jeans, and thongs were never meant to be worn by normal-sized women.

Department store sales clerks are never to be trusted.

Have you ever known one to say "Honey, that outfit makes you look hippy. Why don't you try the store across the mall?"

Shoulder pads never have to go out of style.

Lycra is your friend.

BINGE BYLAWS

If a girlfriend goes on a binge after a bad break-up, you have a moral obligation to join her.

If the break-up wasn't her doing, you are obliged to spring for the ice cream and the liquor.

It is permissible to break a diet when:

There's been a divorce or break-up.

You've been fired.

You've been promoted.

You've paid your rent on time.

Your parents are in town.

Your boyfriend is out of town.

It's Saturday night and you don't have a date.

It's a three-day weekend.

You're dining at a four-star restaurant or above.

You've stuck to the diet for four weeks.

It's Valentine's Day or any other chocolate-oriented holiday.

There's a sale on Ben and Jerry's, Sara Lee, or Russell Stover.

If you eat standing up,
the calories don't count.

*This rule also applies to
anything eaten on your birthday.*

If you are on a business trip with a $100-a-day meal allowance, you may deduct up to $100 worth of calories per diem, excluding liquor.

Likewise, food purchased with a 15 percent off coupon has 15 percent fewer calories.

Silly or improbable food,
like cheese in a can,
has no calories.

*Because who takes food like that
seriously anyway?*

Foods used for medicinal or therapeutic purposes, such as cough drops, hot cocoa, toast, soup and crackers, pizza, or hot fudge sundaes, *don't count.*

Food from the children's menu has 40 percent fewer calories than the same food on the regular menu because it costs 40 percent less.

Food that you eat off other people's plates, especially children's, has no calories. It is "borrowed" food and can thus be "returned."

This is why you can finish your kids' desserts every night without gaining a pound.

Food eaten in total darkness doesn't count.

Eat slowly.

If you can make lunch last eight hours, you won't need dinner.

Broken cookie pieces, brownie crumbs, and slivers of cheesecake contain no calories.

Foods licked off knives, spatulas, or mixer blades have no calories if you are in the act of preparing or cooking food.

The energy you expend while making the food negates any calories contained in the licked portions.

Calorie counts are listed "per serving," meaning from the finished dish; they do not include ingredients while the dish is being prepared.

Likewise, cookie dough and cake batter have no calories until they are baked.

So lick all you want.

Food eaten on the run—
in the car or on foot—
has no calories.

"On the run" is the equivalent of "running," which burns up to eight hundred calories per hour (depending on your weight), thus negating your intake and accelerating your metabolism for the rest of the day.

Hot food that gets cold loses its calories, and they will not be regained when it is reheated if a microwave is used.

If you are eating food sold to you by nonprofit organizations such as the Girl Scouts, high school marching bands, or Little League baseball teams, you may deduct 50 percent of the calories as a charitable donation.

THE NAKED TRUTH (OR FULL DIS-CLOTHES-URE)

―――――♀―――――

Every girl has the right to get dressed in private.

You are never required to stand naked in front of anyone. This includes husbands, boyfriends, and doctors.

Exception: Prison guards, which should be all the motivation you need to stay out of jail.

A naked body looks ten pounds slimmer in the dark.

Subtract five pounds if you are on your back.

Subtract another ten if you are under the covers.

A tan body looks ten pounds slimmer than a pale body.

Never put on a pair of panty hose in front of anyone you're trying to impress.

EXERCISING YOUR RIGHTS

―――♀―――

Sitting is *too* an exercise.

Done properly, it can burn up to thirty calories per hour.

Exercise performed for any charitable cause such as marathons, walkathons, or swimathons burns twice as many calories—one set for you and one for the cause.

Always work out next to people who are in worse shape than you.

You may not interrupt a fellow girl's workout just because you are gasping for breath and need a bagel break.

MIRRORS, SCALES, AND OTHER DISTORTIONS OF NATURE

♀

Weigh yourself once a week—before the weekend, not after.

Don't even think about stepping on a scale when you're suffering from PMS.

What are you, a glutton for punishment?

When your weight fluctuates from one scale to another, even by five pounds or more, the lighter scale is *always* the accurate one.

This is especially important to remember in the gym and at Weight Watchers meetings.

Doctor's office scales always weigh you ten pounds heavier than your real weight.

Department store mirrors
always make you look
ten pounds skinnier
than your mirrors at home.

The camera adds ten pounds.

Fifteen pounds on the beach.

Never permit anyone to take your photo from below chin level.

Never allow anyone to take your photo while you're eating, drinking, squatting, bending over, playing Limbo or Twister, dancing, or jumping into a pool.